Diabetic Tasty Recipes

A Handful of Quick, Delicious Recipes for Your Meals

Roseann Smith

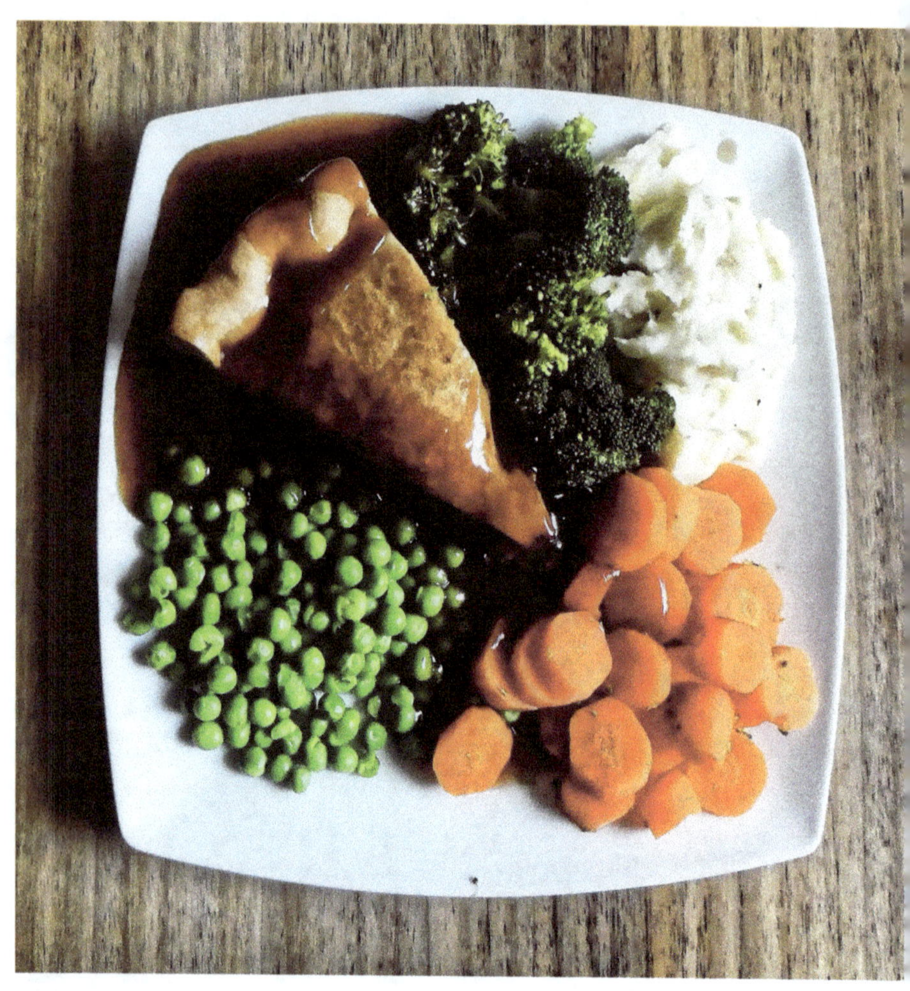

Disclaimer Notice:

Please note the information contained within this document is for educational and entertainment purposes only. All effort has been executed to present accurate, up to date, and reliable, complete information. No warranties of any kind are declared or implied. Readers acknowledge that the author is not engaging in the rendering of legal, financial, medical or professional advice. The content within this book has been derived from various sources. Please consult a licensed professional before attempting any techniques outlined in this book.

By reading this document, the reader agrees that under no circumstances is the author responsible for any losses, direct or indirect, which are incurred as a result of the use of information contained within this document, including, but not limited to, — errors, omissions, or inaccuracies.

Table of Contents

Pork On A Blanket 6

Bacon-wrapped Hot Dog 8

Pork Tenderloin 9

Bacon Cheeseburger Casserole 10

Honey Mustard Pork 12

Barbecue Beef Brisket 13

Cherry Apple Pork 15

Italian Sausage Casserole 17

Pork Fillets With Serrano Ham 18

Maple Glazed Pork 20

Grilled Chicken Wraps 22

Sirloin With Blue Cheese Compound Butter 24

Pork Rind 27

Roasted Pork Shoulder 29

Lamb Curry 31

Mediterranean Lamb Meatballs 34

Irish Pork Roast 36

Vegetables With Irish Beef Roast 38

Rosemary Lamb 40

Roast Pork 42

Marinated Loin Potatoes 43

Curried Lamb On Rice 45

Pork With Pear Stuffing 47

Pork Curry 49

Lamb Chops With Kalamata Tapenade 52

Chicken With Asparagus And Mango 55

Steak With Mushroom Sauce 57

Air Fryer Bacon 59

Chorizo And Beef Burger 60

Lamb & Chickpeas 62

Crunchy Chicken Fingers 64

Polynesian Chicken 66

Buffalo Chicken 68

Chicken & Peanut Stir-fry 70

Meatballs Curry 72

Jerk Style Chicken Wings 76

Italian Chicken 78

Coconut Chicken 80

Spicy Lime Chicken 82

Crock-pot Slow Cooker Ranch Chicken 84

Mustard Chicken With Basil 86

Chicken Chili 88

Chicken With Cashew Nuts 91

Chuck And Veggies 93

Chicken & Broccoli Bake 95

Rosemary Lemon Chicken 98

Ginger Flavored Chicken 100

Crock-pot Slow Cooker Tex-mex Chicken 102

Slow-cooker Chicken Fajita Burritos 104

Chicken With Chickpeas 106

Pork On A Blanket

Servings: 4

Cooking Time: 10 Minutes

Ingredients:

- 1/2 puff defrosted pastry sheet
- 16 thick smoked sausages
- 15 ml of milk

Directions:

1. Adjust the temperature of the air fryer to 200°C and set the timer to 5 minutes.
2. Cut the puff pastry into 64 x 38 mm strips.
3. Place a cocktail sausage at the end of the puff pastry and roll around the sausage, sealing the dough with some water.
4. Brush the top of the sausages wrapped in milk and place them in the preheated air fryer.

5. Cook at 200°C for 10 minutes or until golden brown.

Nutrition Info: Calories: 242 kcal Fat: 14g Carbs: 0g Protein: 27g

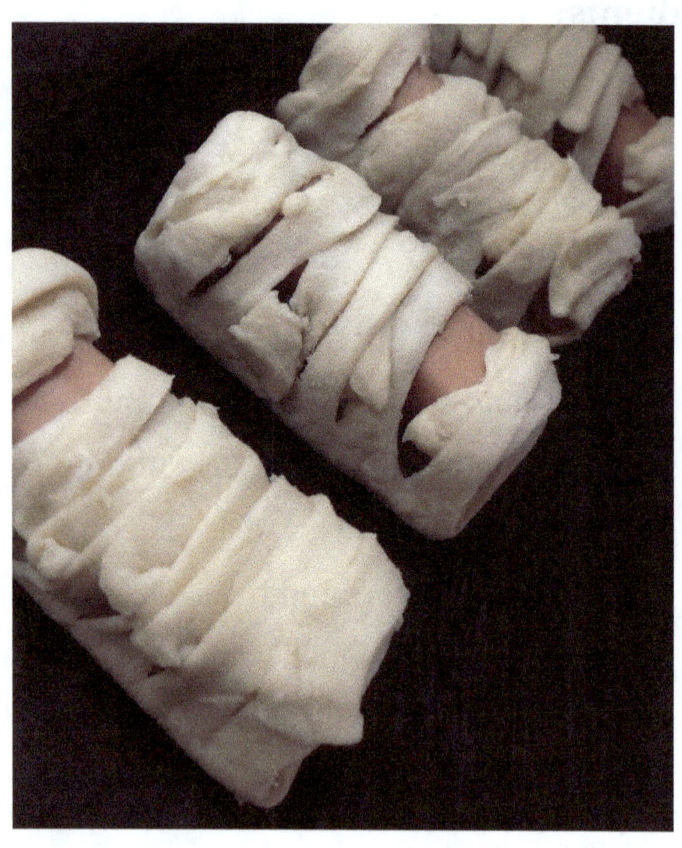

Bacon-wrapped Hot Dog

Servings: 4

Cooking Time: 10 Minutes

Ingredients:

- 4 beef hot dogs
- 4 slices sugar-free bacon

Directions:

1. Wrap each hot dog with slice of bacon and secure with toothpick. Place into the air fryer basket.

2. Adjust the temperature to 370°F and set the timer for 10 minutes.

3. Flip each hot dog halfway through the cooking time. When fully cooked, bacon will be crispy. Serve warm.

Nutrition Info: Calories: 197 Protein: 9.2 G Fiber: 0.0 G Net Carbohydrates: 1.3 G Fat: 15.0 G Sodium: 571 Mg Carbohydrates: 1.3 G Sugar: 0.6 G

Pork Tenderloin

Servings: 6

Cooking Time: 30 Minutes

Ingredients:

- 1-1/2 lbs. pork tenderloin

Directions:

1. Adjust the temperature of the Air Fryer to 370F.
2. Lay the pork in the Air Fryer basket.
3. Cook at 400F for about 30 minutes, turning halfway through cooking time for a proper cook.
4. Serve.

Nutrition Info: Calories: 419 kcal; Fat: 3.5g; Carbs: 0g; Proteins: 26g

Bacon Cheeseburger Casserole

Servings: 4

Cooking Time: 20 Minutes

Ingredients:

- 1 pound 80/20 ground beef
- ¼ medium white onion, peeled and chopped
- 1 cup shredded Cheddar cheese, divided
- 1 large egg
- 4 slices sugar-free bacon, cooked and crumbled
- 2 pickle spears, chopped

Directions:

1. Brown the ground beef in a medium skillet over medium heat about 7–10 minutes. When no pink remains, drain the fat. Remove from heat and add ground beef to large mixing bowl.

2.   Add onion, ½ cup Cheddar, and egg to bowl. Mix ingredients well and add crumbled bacon.

3.   Pour the mixture into a 4-cup round baking dish and top with remaining Cheddar. Place into the air fryer basket.

4.   Adjust the temperature to 375°F and set the timer for 20 minutes.

5.   Casserole will be golden on top and firm in the middle when fully cooked. Serve immediately with chopped pickles on top.

Nutrition Info: Calories: 369 Protein: 31.0 G Fiber: 0.2 G Net Carbohydrates: 1.0 G Fat: 22.6 G Sodium: 454 Mg Carbohydrates: 1.2 G Sugar: 0.5 G

Honey Mustard Pork

Servings: 2

Cooking Time: 60 Minutes

Ingredients:

- 1.5lb rolled, trimmed pork joint
- 1 cup honey mustard sauce, low carb
- salt and pepper

Directions:

1. Mix all the ingredients in your Instant Pot.
2. Cook on Stew for 60 minutes.
3. Release the pressure naturally.

Nutrition Info: Calories: 290 Carbs: 9 Sugar: 8 Fat: 17 Protein: 39 GL: 4

Barbecue Beef Brisket

Servings: 10

Cooking Time: 10 Hours

Ingredients:

- 4 lb. beef brisket (boneless), trimmed and sliced
- 1 bay leaf
- 2 onions, sliced into rings
- ½ teaspoon dried thyme, crushed
- ¼ cup chili sauce
- 1 clove garlic, minced
- Salt and pepper to taste
- 2 tablespoons light brown sugar
- 2 tablespoons cornstarch
- 2 tablespoons cold water

Directions:

1. Put the meat in a slow cooker.
2. Add the bay leaf and onion.

3.   In a bowl, mix the thyme, chili sauce, salt, pepper and sugar.

4.   Pour the sauce over the meat.

5.   Mix well.

6.   Seal the pot and cook on low heat for 10 hours.

7.   Discard the bay leaf.

8.   Pour cooking liquid in a pan.

9.   Add the mixed water and cornstarch.

10.   Simmer until the sauce has thickened.

11. Pour the sauce over the meat.

Nutrition Info: Calories 182 Total Fat 6 g Saturated Fat 2 g Cholesterol 57 mg Sodium 217 mg Total Carbohydrate 9 g Dietary Fiber 1 g Total Sugars 4 g Protein 20 g Potassium 383 mg

Cherry Apple Pork

Servings: 2

Cooking Time: 40 Minutes

Ingredients:

- Apple (1 small, diced)
- Cherries (.3 c pitted)
- Onion (3 T diced)
- Celery (3 T diced)
- Apple juice (.25 c)
- Black pepper
- Pork loin (.75 lb.)
- Water (.25 c)

Directions:

1. Add all of the ingredients to the Instant Pot cooker and mix thoroughly.
2. Seal the lid of the cooker, choose the poultry setting and set the time for 5 minutes.
3. Once the timer goes off, select the quick pressure release option and remove the lid as soon as the pressure has normalized.

4.   Serve warm.

Nutrition Info: Protein: 12 grams Carbs: 22.9 grams Fiber: 19 grams Sugar: 11.2 grams Fats: 28 grams Calories: 453

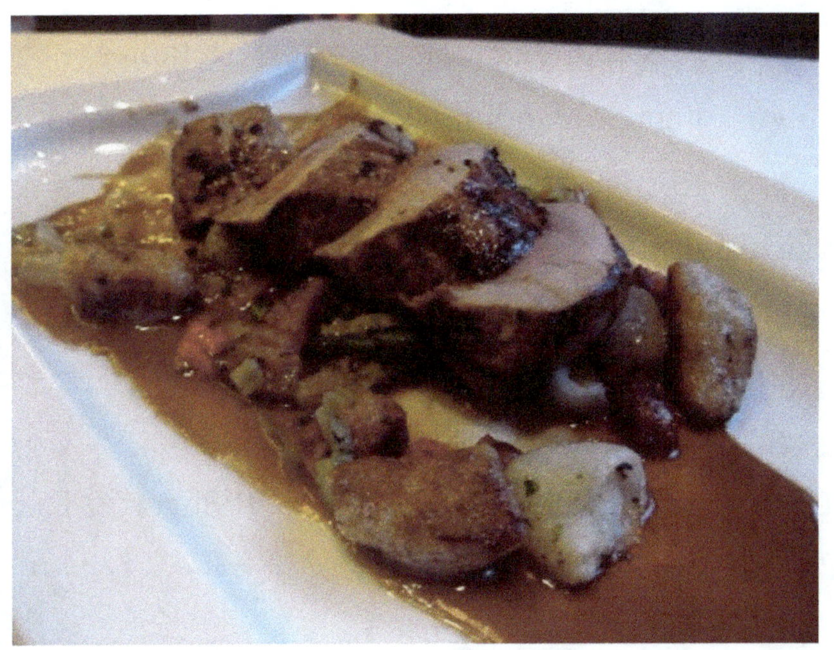

Italian Sausage Casserole

Servings: 2

Cooking Time: 5 Minutes

Ingredients:

- 1lb chopped cooked sausages
- 1lb chopped Mediterranean vegetables
- 1 cup low sodium broth
- 1tbsp mixed herbs

Directions:

1. Mix all the ingredients in your Instant Pot.
2. Cook on Stew for 5 minutes.
3. Release the pressure naturally.

Nutrition Info: Calories: 320 Carbs: 8 Sugar: 2 Fat: 18 Protein: 41 GL: 4

Pork Fillets With Serrano Ham

Servings: 4

Cooking Time: 20 Minutes

Ingredients:

- 400g of very thin sliced pork fillets
- 2 boiled and chopped eggs
- 100g chopped Serrano ham
- 1 beaten egg
- Breadcrumbs

Directions:

1. Make a roll with the pork fillets. Introduce half-cooked egg and Serrano ham. So that the roll does not lose its shape, fasten with a string or chopsticks.

2. Pass the rolls through the beaten egg and then through the breadcrumbs until it forms a good layer.

3. Adjust the temperature of the air fryer for a few minutes at 180° C.

4.   Insert the rolls in the basket and set the timer for about 8 minutes at 180° C.

5.   Serve.

Nutrition Info: Calories: 424 kcal Fat: 15.15g Carbs: 37.47g Protein: 31.84g

Maple Glazed Pork

Servings: 2

Cooking Time: 15 Minutes

Ingredients:

- Maple syrup (.25 c)
- Honey (.25 c)
- Cinnamon (1 tsp)
- Brown sugar (.25 c)
- Orange juice (2 T)
- Nutmeg (1 tsp)
- Bone in ham (1 small)

Directions:

1. Combine everything except for the ham in a saucepan on medium heat; mix well.
2. Put the ham in the cooker. Cook 15 minutes, then use quick release.

3. Set the ham in the baking dish. Pour glaze over ham.

4. Place the ham under a broiler to caramelize the sugars and form a slight char.

Nutrition Info: Protein: 23.8 grams Carbs: 37.5 grams Fiber: 32.8 grams Sugar: 18.2 grams Fats: 42 grams Calories: 540

Grilled Chicken Wraps

Servings: 4

Cooking Time: 6 Minutes

Ingredients:

- 4 oz. chicken breasts, boneless and skinless
- 2 teaspoons oregano, crushed
- ¼ cup mint, chopped
- 2 onion slices, peeled
- What you will need from the store cupboard:
- 2 12-inch Arabic bread or Naan pieces
- 2 tablespoons of lemon juice
- Cooking spray
- Pepper and salt to taste

Directions:

1. Preheat your oven to 350 °F.
2. Brush both sides of the chicken breasts with lemon juice.
3. Sprinkle oregano.

4. Apply cooking spray lightly and return to the grill.

5. Keep the onion slices and chicken breasts on the grill.

6. Cook each side for 3 minutes. Turn once.

7. Cut the onion into strips.

8. Cut the chicken into small ½ strips after it is done.

9. Cut your Arabic bread into half. Leave the pita bread or naan whole.

10. Now keep the onion strips and chicken at the center of the bread pieces.

11. Sprinkle mint. Roll up.

Nutrition Info: Calories 328, Carbohydrates 36g, Fiber 5g, Cholesterol 82mg, Total Fat 3g, Protein 39g, Sodium 415mg

Sirloin With Blue Cheese Compound Butter

Servings: 4

Cooking Time: 12 Minutes

Ingredients:

- 6 tablespoons butter, at room temperature
- 4 ounces' blue cheese, such as Stilton or Roquefort
- 4 (5-ounce) beef sirloin steaks
- 1 tablespoon olive oil
- Sea salt
- Freshly ground black pepper

Directions:

1. Place the butter in a blender and pulse until the butter is whipped, about 2 minutes.

2. Add the cheese and pulse until just incorporated.

3. Spoon the butter mixture onto a sheet of plastic wrap and roll it into a log about 1½ inches in diameter by twisting both ends of the plastic wrap in opposite directions.

4. Refrigerate the butter until completely set, about 1 hour.

5. Slice the butter into ½-inch disks and set them on a plate in the refrigerator until you are ready to serve the steaks. Store leftover butter in the refrigerator for up to 1 week.

6. Preheat a barbecue to medium-high heat.

7. Let the steaks come to room temperature.

8. Rub the steaks all over with the olive oil and season them with salt and pepper.

9. Grill the steaks until they reach your desired doneness, about 6 minutes per side for medium.

10. If you do not have a barbecue, broil the steaks in a preheated oven for 7 minutes per side for medium.

11. Let the steaks rest for 10 minutes. Serve each topped with a disk of the compound butter.

Nutrition Info: Calories: 544 Fat: 44g Protein: 35g Carbs: 0g Fiber: 0g Net Carbs: 0g Fat 72%/Protein 28%/Carbs 0%

Pork Rind

Servings: 4

Cooking Time: 1 Hr

Ingredients:

- 1kg pork rinds
- Salt
- 1/2 tsp black pepper coffee

Directions:

1. Preheat the air fryer. Set the time of 5 minutes and the temperature to 2000C.
2. Cut the bacon into cubes - 1 finger wide.
3. Season with salt and a pinch of pepper.
4. Place in the basket of the air fryer. Set the time of 45 minutes and press the power button.
5. Shake the basket every 10 minutes so that the pork rinds stay golden brown equally.

6.   Once they are ready, drain a little on the paper towel, so they stay dry. Transfer to a plate and serve.

Nutrition Info: Calories: 172 kcal Fat: 10.02g

Carbs: 0g Protein: 19.62g

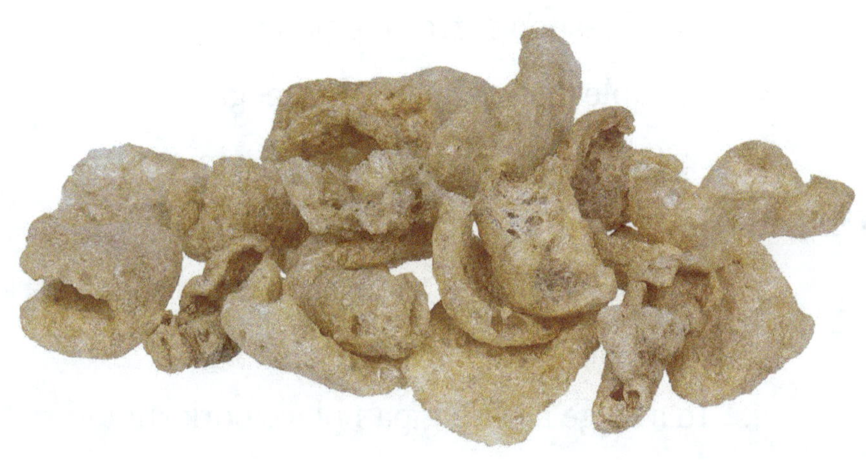

Roasted Pork Shoulder

Servings: 12

Cooking Time: 6 Hours

Ingredients:

- 1 head garlic, peeled and crushed
- ¼ cup fresh rosemary, minced
- 2 tablespoons fresh lemon juice
- 2 tablespoons balsamic vinegar
- 1 (4-pound) pork shoulder, trimmed

Directions:

1. In a bowl, add all the ingredients except pork shoulder and mix well.
2. In a large roasting pan place pork shoulder and coat with marinade generously.
3. With a large plastic wrap, cover the roasting pan and refrigerate to marinate for at least 1-2 hours.
4. Remove the roasting pan from refrigerator.
5. Remove the plastic wrap from roasting pan and keep in room temperature for 1 hour.

6.   Preheat the oven to 275 degrees F.

7.   Arrange the roasting pan in oven and roast for about 6 hours.

8.   Remove from the oven and set aside for about 15-20 minutes.

9.   With a sharp knife, cut the pork shoulder into desired slices and serve.

10.   Meal Prep Tip: Transfer the pork slices onto a wire rack to cool completely. With foil pieces, wrap the pork slices and refrigerate for about 1-2 days. Reheat in the microwave before serving.

Nutrition Info: Calories 450 Total Fat 32.6g Saturated Fat 12 g Cholesterol 136 mg Total Carbs 1.5 g Sugar 0.1 g Fiber 0.6 g Sodium 104 mg Potassium 522 mg Protein 35.4 g

Lamb Curry

Servings: 8

Cooking Time: 2¼ Hours

Ingredients:

- For Spice Mixture:
- 2 teaspoons ground coriander
- 2 teaspoons ground cumin
- 1 teaspoon ground cinnamon
- ½ teaspoon ground ginger
- 1 tablespoons sweet paprika
- ½ tablespoon cayenne pepper
- 1 teaspoon red chili powder
- Salt and ground black pepper, as required
- For Curry:
- 1 tablespoon olive oil
- 2 pounds boneless lamb, trimmed and cubed into 1-inch size
- 2 cups onions, chopped
- ½ cup fat-free plain Greek yogurt, whipped

- 1½ cups water

Directions:

1. For spice mixture: in a bowl, add all spices and mix well. Set aside.
2. In a large Dutch oven, heat the oil over medium-high heat and stir fry the lamb cubes for about 5 minutes.
3. Add the onion and cook for about 4-5 minutes.
4. Stir in the spice mixture and cook for about 1 minute.
5. Add the yogurt and water and bring to a boil over high heat.
6. Now, reduce the heat to low and simmer, covered for about 1-2 hours or until desired doneness of lamb.
7. Uncover and simmer for about 3-4 minutes.
8. Serve hot.
9. Meal Prep Tip: Transfer the curry into a large bowl and set aside to cool. Divide the curry into 8 containers evenly. Cover the

containers and refrigerate for 1-2 days.
Reheat in the microwave before serving.

Nutrition Info: Calories 254 Total Fat 10.5 g Saturated Fat 3.3 g Cholesterol 102 mg Total Carbs 4.7 g Sugar 1.9 g Fiber 1.4 g Sodium 99 mg Potassium 468 mg Protein 34 g

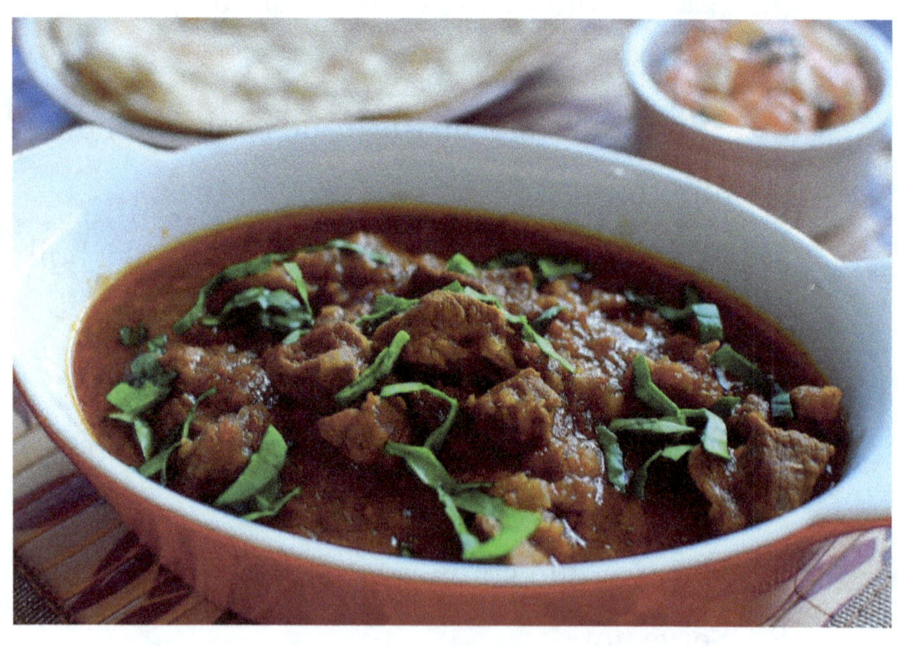

Mediterranean Lamb Meatballs

Servings: 8

Cooking Time: 20 Minutes

Ingredients:

- 12 oz. roasted red peppers
- 1 ½ cups whole wheat breadcrumbs
- 2 eggs, beaten
- 1/3 cup tomato sauce
- ½ cup fresh basil
- ¼ cup parsley, snipped
- Salt and pepper to taste
- 2 lb. lean ground lamb

Directions:

1. Preheat your oven to 350 degrees F.
2. In a bowl, mix all the ingredients and then form into meatballs.
3. Put the meatballs on a baking pan.
4. Bake in the oven for 20 minutes.

Nutrition Info: Calories 94 Total Fat 3 g Saturated Fat 1 g Cholesterol 35 mg Sodium 170 mg Total

Carbohydrate 2 g Dietary Fiber 1 g Total Sugars 0 g
Protein 14 g Potassium 266 mg

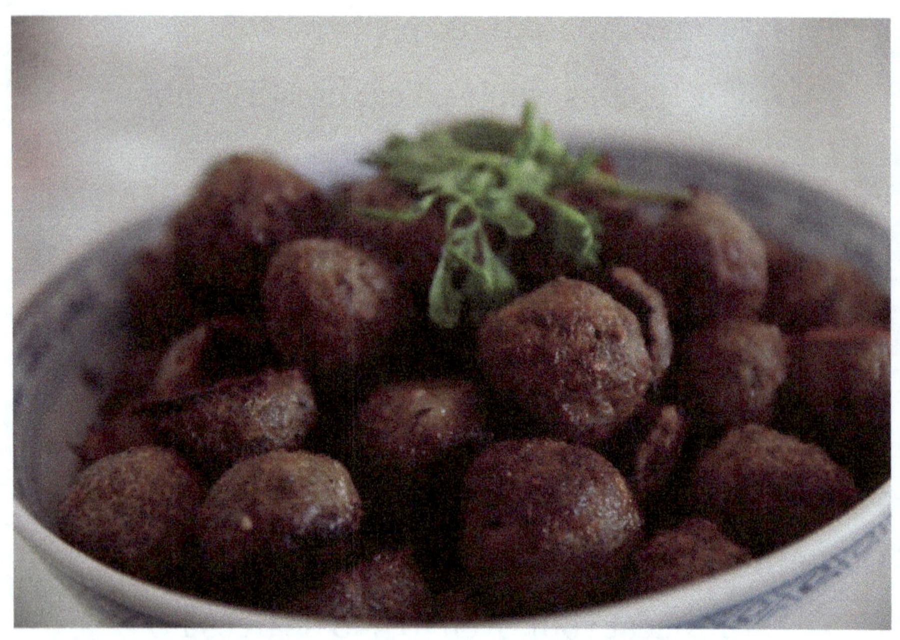

Irish Pork Roast

Servings: 8

Cooking Time: 1 Hour

Ingredients:

- 1 ½ lb. parsnips, peeled and sliced into small pieces
- 1 ½ lb. carrots, sliced into small pieces
- 3 tablespoons olive oil, divided
- 2 teaspoons fresh thyme leaves, divided
- Salt and pepper to taste
- 2 lb. pork loin roast
- 1 teaspoon honey
- 1 cup dry hard cider
- Applesauce

Directions:

1. Preheat your oven to 400 degrees F.
2. Drizzle half of the oil over the parsnips and carrots.
3. Season with half of thyme, salt and pepper.
4. Arrange on a roasting pan.

5. Rub the pork with the remaining oil.

6. Season with the remaining thyme.

7. Season with salt and pepper.

8. Put it on the roasting pan on top of the vegetables.

9. Roast for 65 minutes.

10. Let cool before slicing.

11. Transfer the carrots and parsnips in a bowl and mix with honey.

12. Add the cider.

13. Place in a pan and simmer over low heat until the sauce has thickened.

14. Serve the pork with the vegetables and applesauce.

Nutrition Info: Calories 272 Total Fat 8 g Saturated Fat 2 g Cholesterol 61 mg Sodium 327 mg Total Carbohydrate 23 g Dietary Fiber 6 g Total Sugars 10 g Protein 24 g Potassium 887 mg

Vegetables With Irish Beef Roast

Servings: 8

Cooking Time: 20 Minutes

Ingredients:

- 1 beef rump roast, boneless
- 2 packs mushrooms
- 2 packs (each 1.5 lb.) pot roast vegetables – onions, potatoes, celery, carrots
- 1/3 cup parsley, chopped
- What you will need from the store cupboard:
- 1/3 cup all-purpose flour
- 1 cup beer
- ½ teaspoon black pepper
- ½ teaspoon salt

Directions:

1. Cut the potatoes in half, celery and carrots into 2-inch pieces, and the onions into half-inch wedges. Keep aside.

2.   Bring together the gravy mixes, salt, pepper, and flour in a bowl.

3.   Now add the vegetables to this bowl. Toss for coating.

4.   Take out all vegetables form the flour mix.

5.   Keep in a cooker.

6.   Add the beef roast to bowl. Coat with the flour mixture evenly.

7.   Take out the roast. Keep in the cooker at the center of your vegetables.

8.   Now whisk the beer into the remaining flour mix until it is smooth.

9.   Add to the cooker. Cook covered.

10.   Remove the vegetables and roast.

11. Skim fat from the gravy. Create thin slices from the roast.

12. Serve with gravy and vegetables.

13. If you want, you can sprinkle parsley.

Nutrition Info: Calories 318, Carbohydrates 17g, Cholesterol 112mg, Fat 9g, Fiber 3g, Protein 39g, Sodium 516mg

Rosemary Lamb

Servings: 14

Cooking Time: 2 Hours

Ingredients:

- Salt and pepper to taste
- 2 teaspoons fresh rosemary, snipped
- 5 lb. whole leg of lamb, trimmed and cut with slits on all sides
- 3 cloves garlic, slivered
- 1 cup water

Directions:

1. Preheat your oven to 375 degrees F.
2. Mix salt, pepper and rosemary in a bowl.
3. Sprinkle mixture all over the lamb.
4. Insert slivers of garlic into the slits.
5. Put the lamb on a roasting pan.
6. Add water to the pan.
7. Roast for 2 hours.

Nutrition Info: Calories 136 Total Fat 4 g Saturated Fat 1 g Cholesterol 71 mg Sodium 218 mg Protein 23 g Potassium 248 mg

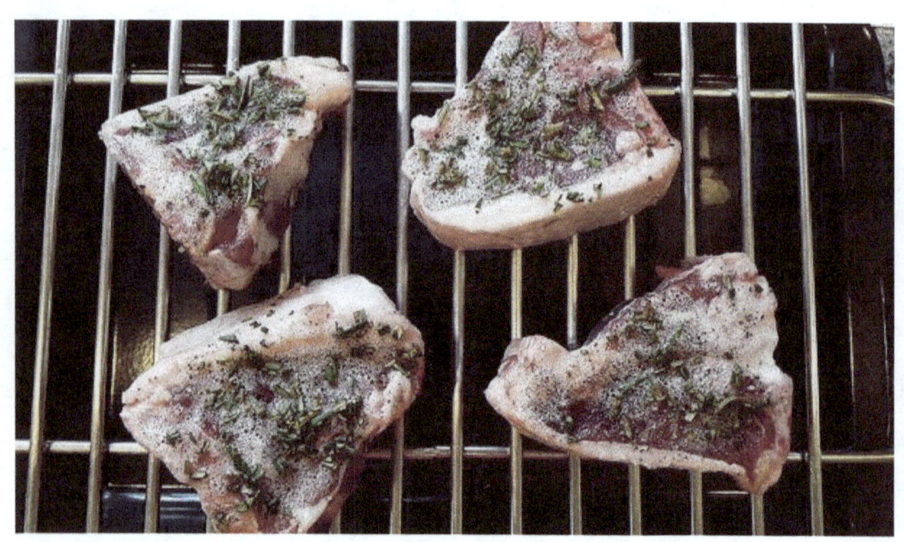

Roast Pork

Servings: 6

Cooking Time: 30 Minutes

Ingredients:

- 2 lbs. pork loin
- 1 Tbsp. olive oil
- 1 tsp. salt

Directions:

1. Adjust the temperature of the Air Fryer to 360F.
2. Apply the oil on the pork.
3. Add salt.
4. Cook the pork in the Air Fryer for about 50 minutes. Shake the food halfway through the cooking
5. Remove the meal from Air Fryer and allow it to cool.
6. Serve

Nutrition Info: Calories: 150 kcal Fat: 6g; Carbs: 0g; Protein: 23.1g

Marinated Loin Potatoes

Servings: 4

Cooking Time: 1 Hr

Ingredients:

- 2 medium potatoes
- 4 fillets of marinated loin
- A little extra virgin olive oil
- Salt

Directions:

1. Peel the potatoes and cut. Cut with matchsized mandolin, potatoes with a cane but very thin.
2. Wash and immerse in water 30 minutes.
3. Drain and dry well.
4. Add a little oil and stir so that the oil permeates well in all the potatoes.
5. Go to the basket of the air fryer and distribute well.

6. Cook at 1600C for 10 minutes.

7. Take out the basket, shake so that the potatoes take off. Let the potato tender. If it is not, leave 5 more minutes.

8. Place the steaks on top of the potatoes.

9. Select, 10 minutes, and 1800C for 5 minutes again.

Nutrition Info: Calories: 136 kcal Fat: 5.1g Carbs: 1.9g Protein: 20.7g

Curried Lamb On Rice

Servings: 4

Cooking Time: 20 Minutes

Ingredients:

- 1 lb. lean lamb, trimmed and cubed
- ¼ teaspoon ginger, ground
- 1 tomato, peeled, seeded and chopped
- ½ cup carrot, grated
- ½ cup onion, chopped
- What you will need from the store cupboard:
- 2 cups of cooked rice
- 1 cup beef broth
- 1 tablespoon margarine
- ¾ teaspoon salt
- 2 teaspoons of curry powder
- 1-1/2 tablespoons all-purpose flour

Directions:

1. Heat a skillet and brown the onion and lamb for 5 minutes in the margarine.
2. Add the curry powder, broth, flour, tomato, and salt. Mix well by stirring.
3. Simmer until the lamb has become tender. Add some water and keep stirring.
4. Now toss the carrot with your rice in a saucepan. Heat.
5. Divide your rice among the serving plates. Place lamb over the rice.

Nutrition Info: Calories 331, Carbohydrates 31g, Fiber 2g, Cholesterol 75mg, Fat 10g, Protein 28g, Sugar 1g

Pork With Pear Stuffing

Servings: 4

Cooking Time: 20 Minutes

Ingredients:

- 1 pork tenderloin
- ¼ cup carrot, shredded
- ½ cup pear, chopped
- 2 tablespoons onion, chopped
- ½ cup pear, chopped
- What you will need from the store cupboard:
- 1 teaspoon cooking oil
- ¼ cup soft breadcrumbs
- 2 tablespoons orange marmalade, sugar-free
- ¼ teaspoon pepper
- ¼ teaspoon salt

Directions:

1.   For the stuffing, bring together the breadcrumbs, pear, onion, pepper, and salt in a bowl. Keep this aside.
2.   Trim fat from the meat. Cut lengthwise down the center.
3.   Open flat. Pound the flat side.
4.   Now spread stuffing over your meat. Fold in the ends. Roll up.
5.   Use wooden toothpicks or kitchen string to secure.
6.   Keep meat roll in your roasting pan.
7.   Brush oil lightly.
8.   Roast for 12 minutes.
9.   Brush some orange marmalade over the meat's top.
10.   Roast again for 3 minutes.

Nutrition Info: Calories 191, Carbohydrates 9g, Fiber 2g, Cholesterol 55mg, Fat 9g, Sugar 0.3g, Protein 20g, Sodium 193mg

Pork Curry

Servings: 2

Cooking Time: 20 Minutes

Ingredients:

- Carrots (2 sliced)
- Turmeric (.25 tsp.)
- Garam masala (1.5 T)
- Diced tomatoes (4 oz.)
- Zucchini (.25 diced)
- Ghee (1 T)
- Black pepper (1 pinch)
- Coconut milk (.5 c)
- Onion (.5 diced)
- Lime juice (.5 limes)
- Ginger (1 inch grated)
- Garlic (2 cloves minced)
- Pork (1 lb.)

Directions:

1. In a sealable container, place the meat before adding in the coconut milk, garlic, lime juice and ginger and mixing thoroughly. Allow the meat to marinate overnight for best results.

2. Place the onions, carrots, garam masala, ghee, tomatoes and meat together in the Instant Pot cooker pot and combine thoroughly.

3. Place the Instant Pot cooker pot into the Instant Pot cooker and seal the lid. Choose the high-pressure option and set the time for 20 minutes.

4. Once the timer goes off, select the natural pressure release option and allow the pot to sit for 10 minutes

5. After opening the lid, switch the Instant Pot cooker to sauté before adding in the zucchini and letting it simmer for 5 minutes.

6. Serve hot over shirataki rice.

Nutrition Info: Protein: 38 grams Carbs: 29 grams Fiber: 23 grams Sugar: 3.5 grams Fats: 33 grams Calories: 520

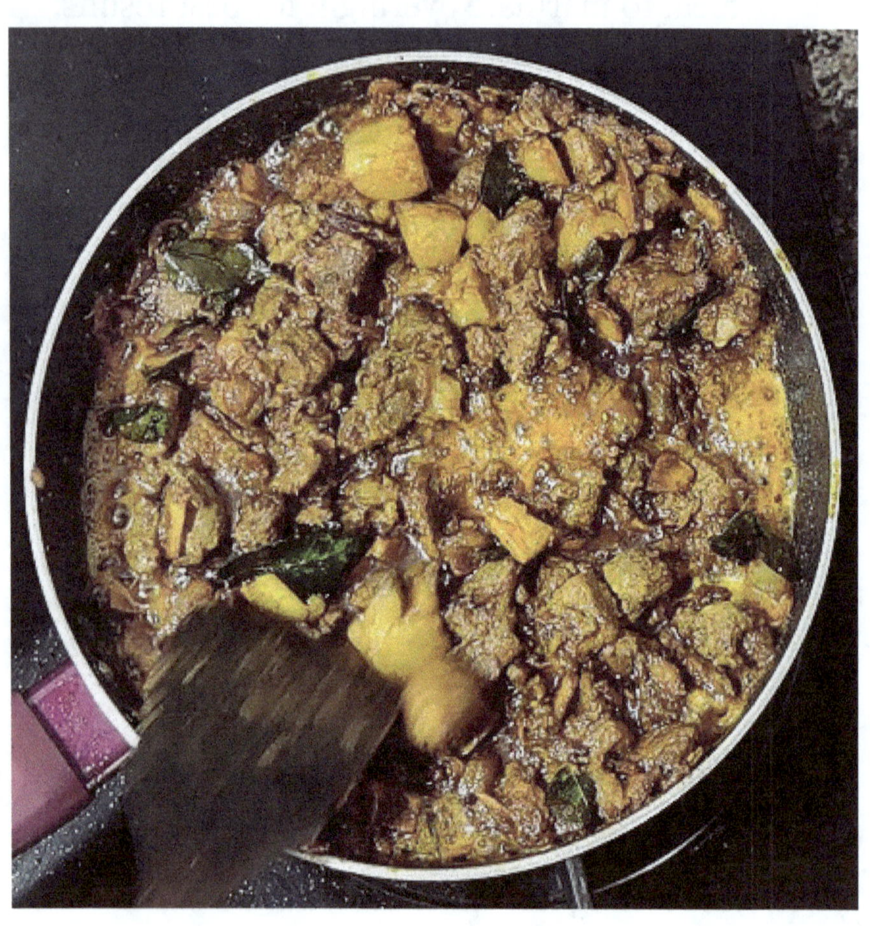

Lamb Chops With Kalamata Tapenade

Servings: 4

Cooking Time: 25 Minutes

Ingredients:

- FOR THE TAPENADE
- 1 cup pitted Kalamata olives
- 2 tablespoons chopped fresh parsley
- 2 tablespoons extra-virgin olive oil
- 2 teaspoons minced garlic
- 2 teaspoons freshly squeezed lemon juice
- FOR THE LAMB CHOPS
- 2 (1-pound) racks French-cut lamb chops (8 bones each)
- Sea salt
- Freshly ground black pepper
- 1 tablespoon olive oil

Directions:

1. Place the olives, parsley, olive oil, garlic, and lemon juice in a food processor and process until the mixture is puréed but still slightly chunky.

2. Transfer the tapenade to a container and store sealed in the refrigerator until needed.

3. TO MAKE THE LAMB CHOPS

4. Preheat the oven to 450°F.

5. Season the lamb racks with salt and pepper.

6. Place a large ovenproof skillet over medium-high heat and add the olive oil.

7. Pan sear the lamb racks on all sides until browned, about 5 minutes in total.

8. Arrange the racks upright in the skillet, with the bones interlaced, and roast them in the oven until they reach your desired doneness, about 20 minutes for medium-rare or until the internal temperature reaches 125°F.

9. Let the lamb rest for 10 minutes and then cut the lamb racks into chops. Arrange 4 chops

per person on the plate and top with the
Kalamata tapenade.

Nutrition Info: Calories: 348 Fat: 28g Protein: 21g
Carbs: 2g Fiber: 1g Net Carbs: 1g Fat 72%/Protein
25%/Carbs 3%

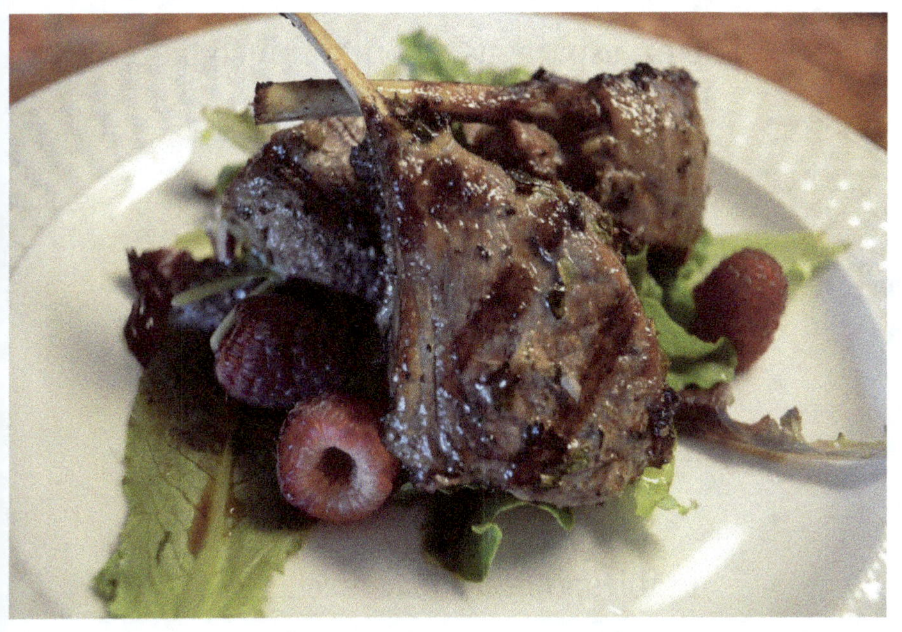

Chicken With Asparagus And Mango

Servings: 4

Cooking Time: 15 Minutes

Ingredients:

- 1 lb. chicken breast, skinless
- 1 ripe mango, peeled, cut into chunks
- 6 oz. asparagus, cut into 2-inch pieces
- 1 egg white
- ½ red bell pepper, seeded
- What you will need from the store cupboard:
- ½ tablespoon canola oil
- 2-1/2 tablespoons vodka
- ½ cup dry white wine
- 1 tablespoon of cornstarch
- 1 tablespoon soy sauce, low-sodium

Directions:

1. Keep the chicken in a bowl.
2. Now add the cornstarch, egg white, canola oil, and vodka. Stir to coat well.
3. Set aside, while preparing the other part of the recipe.
4. Bring together the soy sauce, chicken stock and white wine in your pitcher.
5. Heat your nonstick skillet. Apply cooking oil.
6. Add your marinated chicken. Cook over high temperature until it browns.
7. Add the asparagus and red pepper. Stir fry for 1 minute.
8. Stir the liquid in slowly. Boil to thicken the sauce.
9. Bring down the heat. Stir the mango in.
10. Serve with basmati rice.

Nutrition Info: Calories 213, Carbohydrates 9g, Fiber 2g, Cholesterol 66mg, Total Fat 3g, Protein 29g, Sodium 231mg

Steak With Mushroom Sauce

Servings: 4

Cooking Time: 5 Minutes

Ingredients:

- 12 oz. sirloin steak, sliced and trimmed
- 2 teaspoons grilling seasoning
- 2 teaspoons oil
- 6 oz. broccoli, trimmed
- 2 cups frozen peas
- 3 cups fresh mushrooms, sliced
- 1 cup beef broth (unsalted)
- 1 tablespoon mustard
- 2 teaspoons cornstarch
- Salt to taste

Directions:

1. Preheat your oven to 350 degrees F.
2. Season meat with grilling seasoning.
3. In a pan over medium high heat, cook the meat and broccoli for 4 minutes.
4. Sprinkle the peas around the steak.
5. Put the pan inside the oven and bake for 8 minutes.
6. Remove both meat and vegetables from the pan.
7. Add the mushrooms to the pan.
8. Cook for 3 minutes.
9. Mix the broth, mustard, salt and cornstarch.
10. Add to the mushrooms.
11. Cook for 1 minute.
12. Pour sauce over meat and vegetables before serving.

Nutrition Info: Calories 226 Total Fat 6 g Saturated Fat 2 g Cholesterol 51 mg Sodium 356 mg Total Carbohydrate 16 g Dietary Fiber 5 g Total Sugars 6 g Protein 26 g Potassium 780 mg

Air Fryer Bacon

Servings: 4

Cooking Time: 10 Minutes

Ingredients:

- 11 slices bacon

Directions:

1. Divide the bacon in half, and place the first half in the air fryer.

2. Set the temperature at 401 degrees F, and set the timer to 11 mins.

3. Check it halfway through to see if anything needs to be rearranged.

4. Cook remainder of the time. Serve.

Nutrition Info: Calories: 91 kcal Carbs: 0g Protein: 2g Fat: 8g

Chorizo And Beef Burger

Servings: 4

Cooking Time: 15 Minutes

Ingredients:

- ¾ pound 80/20 ground beef
- ¼ pound Mexican-style ground chorizo
- ¼ cup chopped onion
- 5 slices pickled jalapeños, chopped
- 2 teaspoons chili powder
- 1 teaspoon minced garlic
- ¼ teaspoon cumin

Directions:

1. In a large bowl, mix all ingredients. Divide the mixture into four sections and form them into burger patties.
2. Place burger patties into the air fryer basket, working in batches if necessary.
3. Adjust the temperature to 375°F and set the timer for 15 minutes.

4. Flip the patties halfway through the cooking time. Serve warm.

Nutrition Info: Calories: 291 Protein: 21.6 G Fiber: 0.9 G Net Carbohydrates: 3.8 G Fat: 18.3 G Sodium: 474 Mg Carbohydrates: 4.7 G Sugar: 2.5 G

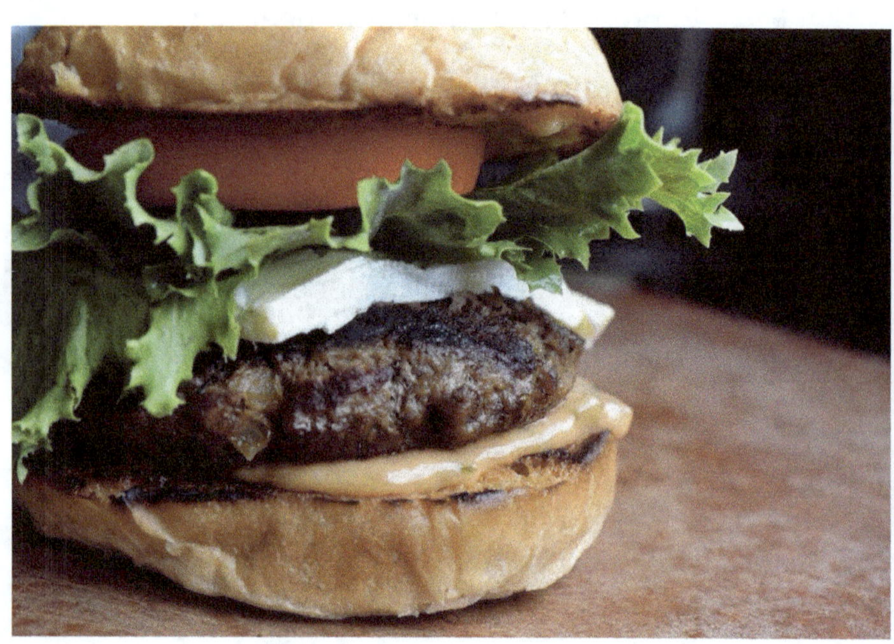

Lamb & Chickpeas

Servings: 4

Cooking Time: 30 Minutes

Ingredients:

- 1 lb. lamb leg (boneless), trimmed and sliced into small pieces
- 2 tablespoons olive oil
- 1 teaspoon ground coriander
- Salt and pepper to taste
- ½ teaspoon ground cumin
- ¼ teaspoon red pepper, crushed
- ¼ cup fresh mint, chopped
- 2 teaspoons lemon zest
- 2 cloves garlic, minced
- 30 oz. unsalted chickpeas, rinsed and drained
- 1 cup tomatoes, chopped
- 1 cup English cucumber, chopped
- ¼ cup fresh parsley, snipped

- 1 tablespoon red wine vinegar

Directions:

1. Preheat your oven to 375 degrees F.
2. Place the lamb on a baking dish.
3. Toss in half of the following: oil, cumin and coriander.
4. Season with red pepper, salt and pepper.
5. Mix well.
6. Roast for 20 minutes.
7. In a bowl, combine the rest of the ingredients with the remaining seasonings.
8. Add salt and pepper.
9. Serve lamb with chickpea mixture.

Nutrition Info: Calories 366 Total Fat 15 g Saturated Fat 3 g Cholesterol 74 mg Sodium 369 mg Total Carbohydrate 27 g Dietary Fiber 7 g Total Sugars 3 g Protein 32 g Potassium 579 mg

Crunchy Chicken Fingers

Servings: 2

Cooking Time: 4 Minutes

Ingredients:

- 2 medium-sized chicken breasts, cut in stripes
- 3 tbsp parmesan cheese
- ¼ tbsp fresh chives, chopped
- ⅓ cup breadcrumbs
- 1 egg white
- 2 tbsp plum sauce, optional
- ½ tbsp fresh thyme, chopped
- ½ tbsp black pepper
- 1 tbsp water

Directions:

1. Preheat the Air Fryer to 360 F. Mix the chives, parmesan, thyme, pepper and breadcrumbs. In another bowl, whisk the egg white and mix with the water. Dip the chicken strips into the egg mixture and the

breadcrumb mixture. Place the strips in the
air fryer basket and cook for 10 minutes.
Serve with plum sauce.

Nutrition Info: Calories: 253; Carbs: 31g; Fat: 18g;
Protein: 28g

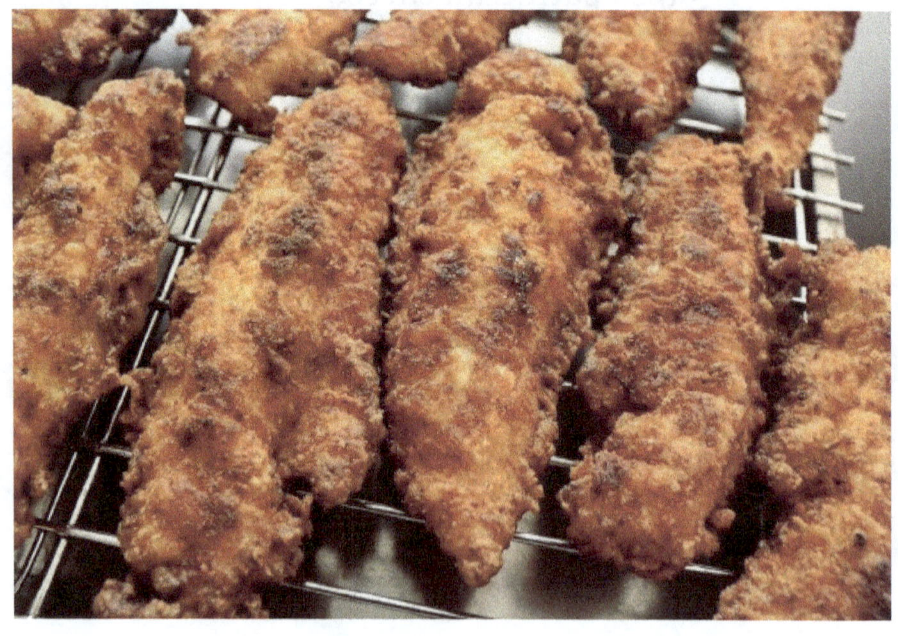

Polynesian Chicken

Servings: 6 Cups

Cooking Time: 4 Hours

Ingredients:

- 3 garlic cloves, minced

- 2 bell peppers, cut into 1/2-inch strips

- 1 (20-ounce) can pineapple chunks in juice, drained, with juice reserved

- 1 1/2-pound boneless chicken breasts, cut into 2-inch cubes

- 1/3 cup honey

- 2 tablespoons tapioca flour

- 3 tablespoons low-sodium soy sauce

- 1 teaspoon ground ginger

Directions:

1. Add reserved pineapple juice, 3 tablespoons of soy sauce, 1/3 cup honey, 1 teaspoon ground ginger and 3 minced cloves of garlic into a bowl; whisk well. Then add 2

tablespoons tapioca flour and whisk again
until combined.

2. Add chicken along with chunks of pineapple
into a slow cooker.

3. Pour mixture of pineapple juice over chicken
and cover the cooker.

4. Cook for about 4-5 hours on low, until
chicken is completely cooked through.

5. Then add strips of bell pepper in the last
hour of cooking. Serve and enjoy!

Nutrition Info: 273 calories; 26 g fat; 37 g total
carbs; 26 g protein

Buffalo Chicken

Servings: 8

Cooking Time: 30 Minutes

Ingredients:

- 2 celery stalks, diced
- 1 medium-sized onion, chopped
- 100 ml buffalo wing sauce
- 100 ml chicken broth
- 21 kg chicken breasts, frozen

Directions:

1. Add the celery, onions, wing sauce, chicken broth and chicken to the Instant Pot. Cook frozen chicken on high pressure for 20 minutes. Turn the pressure valve to "Vent" to release all of the pressure.

2. Remove the chicken breasts from the pot, and shred.

3. You can remove most of the liquid from the
    pot, or not.

Nutrition Info: Calories: 197 Fat: 8g Carbohydrates:
16g Protein: 14g

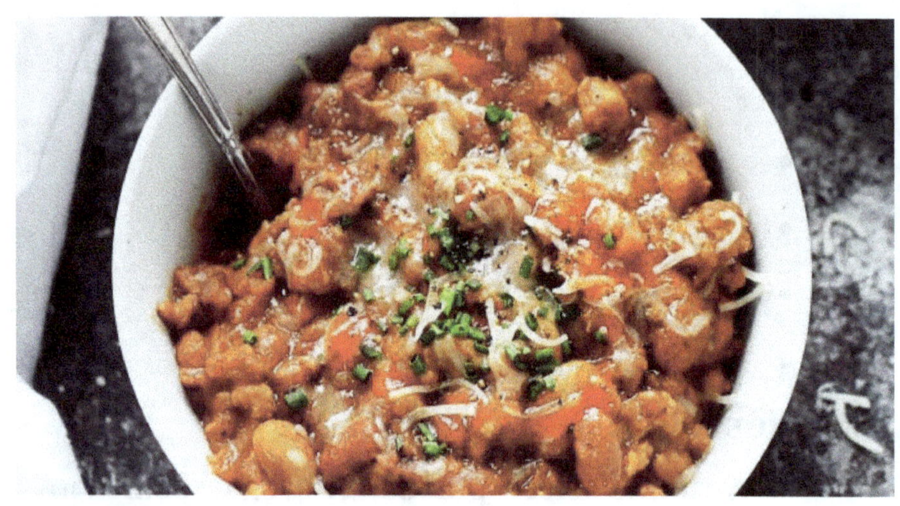

Chicken & Peanut Stir-fry

Servings: 4

Cooking Time: 15 Minutes

Ingredients:

- 3 tablespoons lime juice
- ½ teaspoon lime zest
- 4 cloves garlic, minced
- 2 teaspoons chili bean sauce
- 1 tablespoon fish sauce
- 1 tablespoon water
- 2 tablespoons peanut butter
- 3 teaspoons oil, divided
- 1 lb. chicken breast, sliced into strips
- 1 red sweet pepper, sliced into strips
- 3 green onions, sliced thinly
- 2 cups broccoli, shredded
- 2 tablespoons peanuts, chopped

Directions:

1. In a bowl, mix the lime juice, lime zest, garlic, chili bean sauce, fish sauce, water and peanut butter.
2. Mix well.
3. In a pan over medium high heat, add 2 teaspoons of oil.
4. Cook the chicken until golden on both sides.
5. Pour in the remaining oil.
6. Add the pepper and green onions.
7. Add the chicken, broccoli and sauce.
8. Cook for 2 minutes.
9. Top with peanuts before serving.

Nutrition Info: Calories 368 Total Fat 11 g Saturated Fat 2 g Cholesterol 66 mg Sodium 556 mg Total Carbohydrate 34 g Dietary Fiber 3 g Total Sugars 4 g Protein 32 g Potassium 482 mg

Meatballs Curry

Servings: 6

Cooking Time: 25 Minutes

Ingredients:

- For Meatballs:
- 1 pound lean ground chicken
- 1 tablespoon onion paste
- 1 teaspoons fresh ginger paste
- 1 teaspoons garlic paste
- 1 green chili, chopped finely
- 1 tablespoon fresh cilantro leaves, chopped
- 1 teaspoon ground coriander
- ½ teaspoon cumin seeds
- ½ teaspoon red chili powder
- ½ teaspoon ground turmeric
- 1/8 teaspoon salt
- For Curry:
- 3 tablespoons olive oil
- ½ teaspoon cumin seeds

- 1 (1-inch) cinnamon stick

- 2 onions, chopped

- 1 teaspoons fresh ginger, minced

- 1 teaspoons garlic, minced

- 4 tomatoes, chopped finely

- 2 teaspoons ground coriander

- 1 teaspoon garam masala powder

- ½ teaspoon ground nutmeg

- ½ teaspoon red chili powder

- ½ teaspoon ground turmeric

- Salt, as required

- 1 cup filtered water

- 3 tablespoons fresh cilantro, chopped

Directions:

1. For meatballs: in a large bowl, add all ingredients and mix until well combined.

2. Make small equal-sized meatballs from mixture.

3. In a large deep skillet, heat the oil over medium heat and cook the meatballs for

about 3-5 minutes or until browned from all
sides.

4. Transfer the meatballs into a bowl.

5. In the same skillet, add the cumin seeds and
cinnamon stick and sauté for about 1 minute.

6. Add the onions and sauté for about 4-5
minutes.

7. Add the ginger and garlic paste and sauté for
about 1 minute.

8. Add the tomato and spices and cook,
crushing with the back of spoon for about 2-3
minutes.

9. Add the water and meatballs and bring to a
boil.

10. Now, reduce the heat to low and simmer for
about 10 minutes.

11. Serve hot with the garnishing of cilantro.

12. Meal Prep Tip: Transfer the curry into a large
bowl and set aside to cool. Divide the curry
into 5 containers evenly. Cover the containers
and refrigerate for 1-2 days. Reheat in the
microwave before serving.

Nutrition Info: Calories 196 Total Fat 11.4 g Saturated Fat 2.4 g Cholesterol 53 mg Total Carbs 7.9 g Sugar 3.9 g Fiber 2.1 g Sodium 143 mg Potassium 279 mg Protein 16.7 g

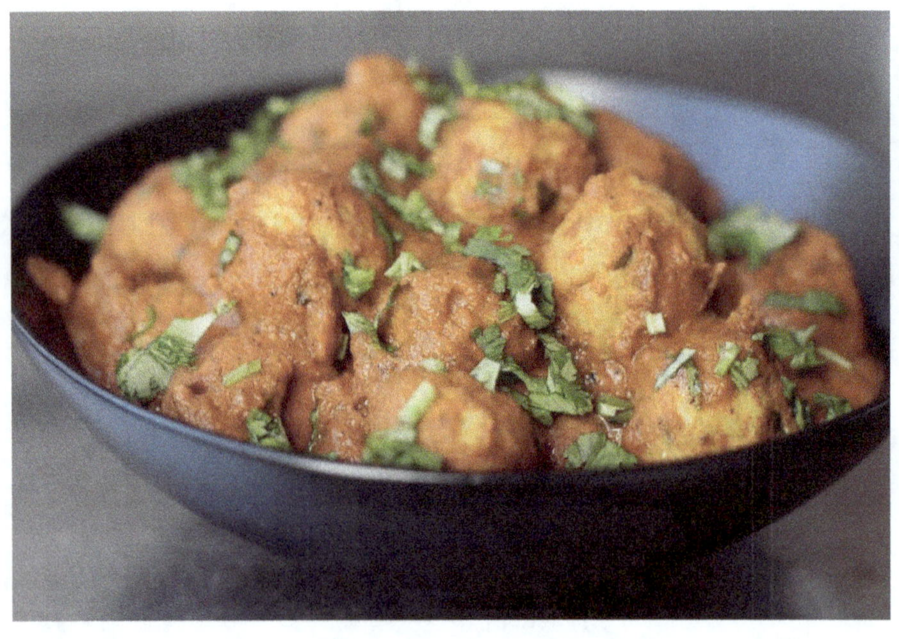

Jerk Style Chicken Wings

Servings: 2-3

Cooking Time: 25 Minutes.

Ingredients:

- 1g ground thyme
- 1g dried rosemary
- 2g allspice
- 4g ground ginger
- 3 g garlic powder
- 2g onion powder
- 1g of cinnamon
- 2g of paprika
- 2g chili powder
- 1g nutmeg
- Salt to taste
- 30 ml of vegetable oil
- 0.5 - 1 kg of chicken wings
- 1 lime, juice

Directions:

1. Select Preheat, set the temperature to 200°C and press Start/Pause.
2. Combine all spices and oil in a bowl to create a marinade.
3. Mix the chicken wings in the marinade until they are well covered.
4. Place the chicken wings in the preheated air fryer.
5. Select Chicken and press Start/Pause. Be sure to shake the baskets in the middle of cooking.
6. Remove the wings and place them on a serving plate.
7. Squeeze fresh lemon juice over the wings and serve.

Nutrition Info: Calories: 240 Fat: 15g Carbohydrate: 5g Protein: 19g Sugars: 4g Cholesterol: 60mg

Italian Chicken

Servings: 4

Cooking Time: 16 Minutes

Ingredients:

- 5 chicken thighs
- 1 tbsp. olive oil
- 1/4 cup parmesan; grated
- 1/2 cup sun dried tomatoes
- 2 garlic cloves; minced
- 1 tbsp. thyme; chopped.
- 1/2 cup heavy cream
- 3/4 cup chicken stock
- 1 tsp. red pepper flakes; crushed
- 2 tbsp. basil; chopped
- Salt and black pepper to the taste

Directions:

1. Season chicken with salt and pepper, rub with half of the oil, place in your preheated air fryer at 350 °F and cook for 4 minutes.

2. Meanwhile; heat up a pan with the rest of the oil over medium high heat, add thyme garlic, pepper flakes, sun dried tomatoes, heavy cream, stock, parmesan, salt and pepper; stir, bring to a simmer, take off heat and transfer to a dish that fits your air fryer.

3. Add chicken thighs on top, introduce in your air fryer and cook at 320 °F, for 12 minutes. Divide among plates and serve with basil sprinkled on top.

Nutrition Info: Calories: 272; Fat: 9; Fiber: 12; Carbs: 37; Protein: 23

Coconut Chicken

Servings: 6

Cooking Time: 4 Hours

Ingredients:

- 2 garlic cloves, minced
- Fresh cilantro, minced
- 1/2 cup light coconut milk
- 6 tablespoons sweetened coconut, shredded and toasted
- 2 tablespoons brown sugar
- 6 (about 1-1/2 pounds) boneless skinless chicken thighs
- 2 tablespoons reduced-sodium soy sauce
- 1/8 teaspoon ground cloves

Directions:

1. Mix brown sugar, 1/2 cup light coconut milk, 2 tablespoons soy sauce, 1/8 teaspoon ground cloves and 2 minced cloves of garlic in a bowl.

2. Add 6 chicken boneless thighs into a Crockpot.

3.   Now pour the mixture of coconut milk over chicken thighs. Cover the cooker and cook for about 4-5 hours on low.

4.   Serve coconut chicken with cilantro and coconut; enjoy!

Nutrition Info: 201 calories; 10 g fat; 6 g total carbs; 21 g protein

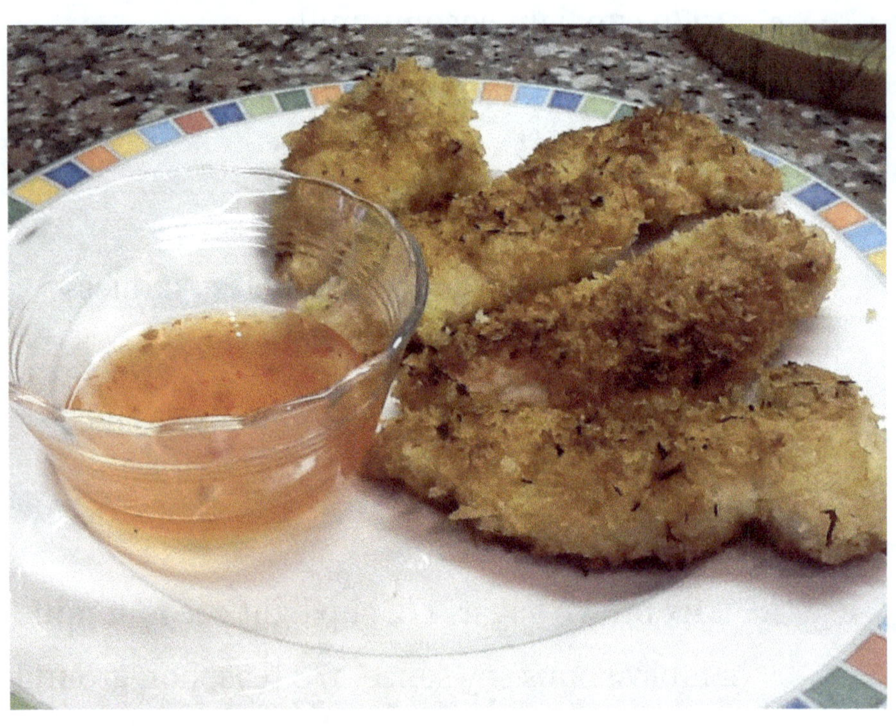

Spicy Lime Chicken

Servings: 6

Cooking Time: 3 Hours

Ingredients:

- 3 tablespoons lime juice
- Fresh cilantro leaves
- 1-1/2 pounds (about 4) boneless skinless chicken breast halves
- 1 teaspoon lime zest, grated
- 2 cups chicken broth
- 1 tablespoon chili powder

Directions:

1. Add chicken breast halves into a slow cooker.
2. Add 1 tablespoon chili powder, 3 tablespoons lime juice and 2 cups chicken broth in a small bowl; mix well and pour over chicken.
3. Cover the cooker and cook for about 3 hours on low. Once done, take chicken out from the cooker and let it cool.

4. Once cooled, shred chicken by using forks and transfer back to the Crockpot.

5. Stir in 1 teaspoon grated lime zest. Serve spicy lime chicken with cilantro and enjoy!

Nutrition Info: 132 calories; 3 g fat; 2 g total carbs; 23 g protein

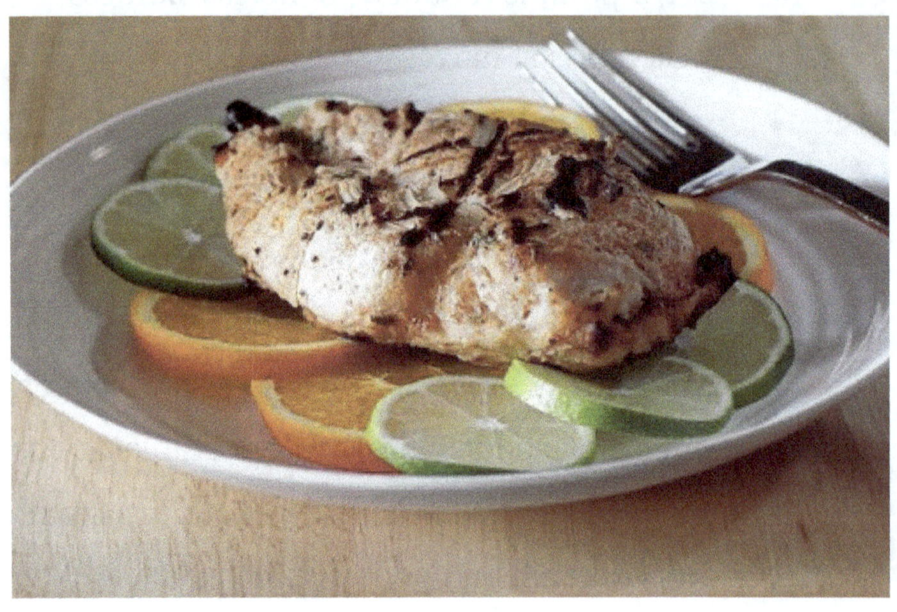

Crock-pot Slow Cooker Ranch Chicken

Servings: 4

Cooking Time: 4 Hours

Ingredients:

- 1 cup chive and onion cream cheese spread
- ½ teaspoon freshly ground black pepper
- 4 boneless chicken breasts
- 1 1-oz package ranch dressing and seasoning mix
- ½ cup low sodium chicken stock

Directions:

1. Spray the Crock-Pot slow cooker with cooking spray and preheat it.
2. Dry chicken with paper towel and transfer it to the Crock-Pot slow cooker.
3. Cook each side, until chicken is browned, for about 4-5 minutes.

4.   Add ½ cup low sodium chicken stock, 1 1-oz.
     package ranch dressing and seasoning mix, 1
     cup chive and onion cream cheese spread and
     ½ teaspoon freshly ground black pepper.
     Cover the Crock-Pot slow cooker and cook for
     about 4 hours on Low or until the internal
     temperature reaches 165 F. Once cooked, take
     it out from the Crock-Pot slow cooker.

5.   Whisk the sauce present in the Crock-Pot
     slow cooker until smooth. If you need thick
     sauce, then cook for about 5-10 minutes, with
     frequent stirring.

6.   Garnish chicken with sliced onions and
     bacon and serve.

Nutrition Info: 362 calories; 18.5 g fat; 9.7 g total
carbs; 37.3 g protein

Mustard Chicken With Basil

Servings: 4

Cooking Time: 30 Minutes

Ingredients:

- 1 tsp Chicken stock
- 2 Chicken breasts; skinless and boneless chicken breasts: halved
- 1 tbsp Chopped basil
- What you'll need from the store cupboard:
- Salt and black pepper
- 1 tbsp Olive oil
- ½ tsp Garlic powder
- ½ tsp Onion powder
- 1 tsp Dijon mustard

Directions:

1. Press 'Sauté' on the instant pot and add the oil. When it is hot, brown the chicken in it for 2-3 minutes.

2.   Mix in the remaining ingredients and seal the lid to cook for 12 minutes at high pressure.

3.   Natural release the pressure for 10 minutes, share into plates and serve.

Nutrition Info: Calories 34, fat 3.6, carbs 0.7, protein 0.3, fiber 0.1

Chicken Chili

Servings: 6

Cooking Time: 40 Minutes

Ingredients:

- 4 cups low-sodium chicken broth, divided
- 3 cups boiled black beans, divided
- 1 tablespoon extra-virgin olive oil
- 1 large onion, chopped
- 1 jalapeño pepper, seeded and chopped
- 4 garlic cloves, minced
- 1 teaspoon dried thyme, crushed
- 1½ tablespoons ground coriander
- 1 tablespoon ground cumin
- ½ tablespoon red chili powder
- 4 cups cooked chicken, shredded
- 1 tablespoon fresh lime juice
- ¼ cup fresh cilantro, chopped

Directions:

1. In a food processor, add 1 cup of broth and 1 can of black beans and pulse until smooth.
2. Transfer the beans puree into a bowl and set aside.
3. In a large pan, heat the oil over medium heat and sauté the onion and jalapeño for about 4-5 minutes.
4. Add the garlic, spices and sea salt and sauté for about 1 minute.
5. Add the beans puree and remaining broth and bring to a boil.
6. Now, reduce the heat to low and simmer for about 20 minutes.
7. Stir in the remaining can of beans, chicken and lime juice and bring to a boil.
8. Now, reduce the heat to low and simmer for about 5-10 minutes.
9. Serve hot with the garnishing of cilantro.
10. Meal Prep Tip: Transfer the chili into a large bowl and set aside to cool. Divide the chili into 6 containers evenly. Cover the

containers and refrigerate for 1-2 days.

Reheat in the microwave before serving.

Nutrition Info: Calories 356 Total Fat 7.1 g Saturated Fat 1.2 g Cholesterol 72 mg Total Carbs 33 g Sugar 2.7 g Fiber 11.6 g Sodium 130 mg Potassium 662 mg Protein 39.6 g

Chicken With Cashew Nuts

Servings: 4

Cooking Time: 30 Minutes

Ingredients:

- 1 lb chicken cubes
- 2 tbsp soy sauce
- 1 tbsp corn flour
- 2 ½ onion cubes
- 1 carrot, chopped
- ⅓ cup cashew nuts, fried
- 1 capsicum, cut
- 2 tbsp garlic, crushed
- Salt and white pepper

Directions:

1. Marinate the chicken cubes with ½ tbsp of white pepper, ½ tsp salt, 2 tbsp soya sauce, and add 1 tbsp corn flour.
2. Set aside for 25 minutes. Preheat the Air Fryer to 380 F and transfer the marinated chicken. Add the garlic, the onion, the

capsicum, and the carrot; fry for 5-6 minutes.

Roll it in the cashew nuts before serving.

Nutrition Info: Calories: 425; Carbs: 25g; Fat: 35g; Protein: 53g

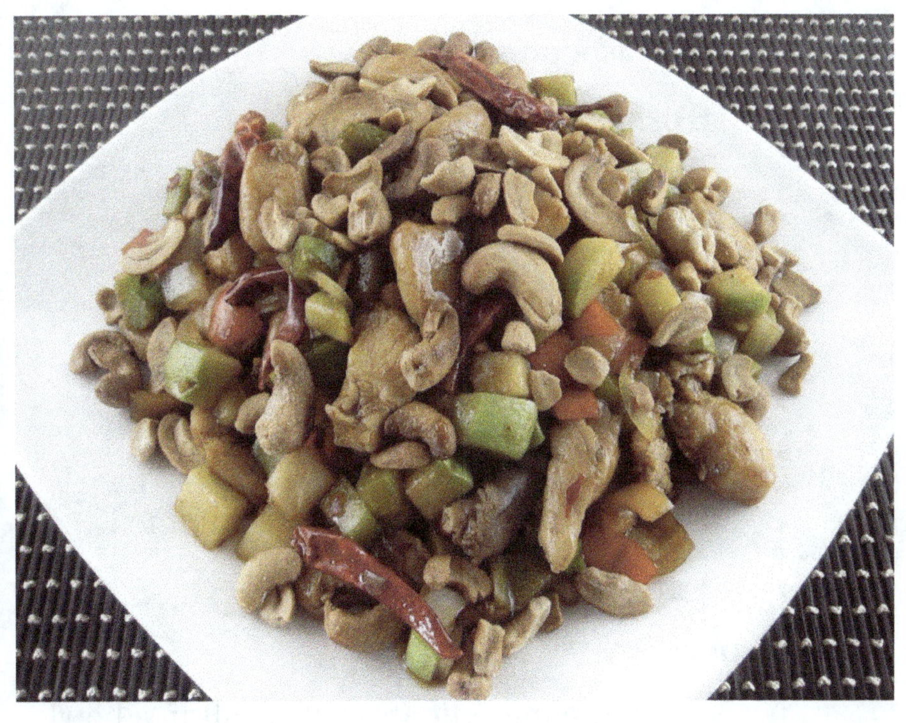

Chuck And Veggies

Servings: 2

Cooking Time: 9 Hours

Ingredients:

- ¼ cup dry red wine
- ¼ teaspoon salt
- 8 oz. boneless lean chuck roast
- ¼ teaspoon black pepper
- 8 oz. frozen pepper stir-fry
- 1 teaspoon Worcestershire sauce
- 8 oz. whole mushrooms
- 1 teaspoon instant coffee granules
- 1 1/4 cups fresh green beans, trimmed
- 1 dried bay leaf

Directions:

1. Mix all the ingredients except salt in a bowl; combine well and then transfer to a slow cooker.

2.   Cover the cooker and cook for about 9 hours on low and 4 1/2 hours on high, until beef is completely cooked through and tender.

3.   Stir in ¼ teaspoon salt gently. Take out the vegetables and beef and transfer to 2 shallow bowls.

4.   Pour liquid into the skillet; boil it lightly and cook until liquid reduces to ¼ cup, for about 1 1/2 minutes.

5.   Pour over veggies and beef. Discard bay leaf and serve.

Nutrition Info: 215 calories; 5 g fat; 17 g total carbs; 26 g protein

Chicken & Broccoli Bake

Servings: 6

Cooking Time: 45 Minutes

Ingredients:

- 6 (6-ounce) boneless, skinless chicken breasts
- 3 broccoli heads, cut into florets
- 4 garlic cloves, minced
- ¼ cup olive oil
- 1 teaspoon dried oregano, crushed
- 1 teaspoon dried rosemary, crushed
- Sea Salt and ground black pepper, as required

Directions:

1. Preheat the oven to 375 degrees F. Grease a large baking dish.
2. In a large bowl, add all the ingredients and toss to coat well.

3. In the bottom of prepared baking dish, arrange the broccoli florets and top with chicken breasts in a single layer.

4. Bake for about 45 minutes.

5. Remove from the oven and set aside for about 5 minutes before serving.

6. Meal Prep Tip: Remove the baking dish from the oven and set aside to cool completely. In 6 containers, divide the chicken breasts and broccoli evenly and refrigerate for about 2 days. Reheat in microwave before serving.

Nutrition Info: Calories 443 Total Fat 21.5 g Saturated Fat 4.7 g Cholesterol 151 mg Total Carbs 9.4 g Sugar 2.2g Fiber 3.6 g Sodium 189 mg Potassium 831 mg Protein 53 g

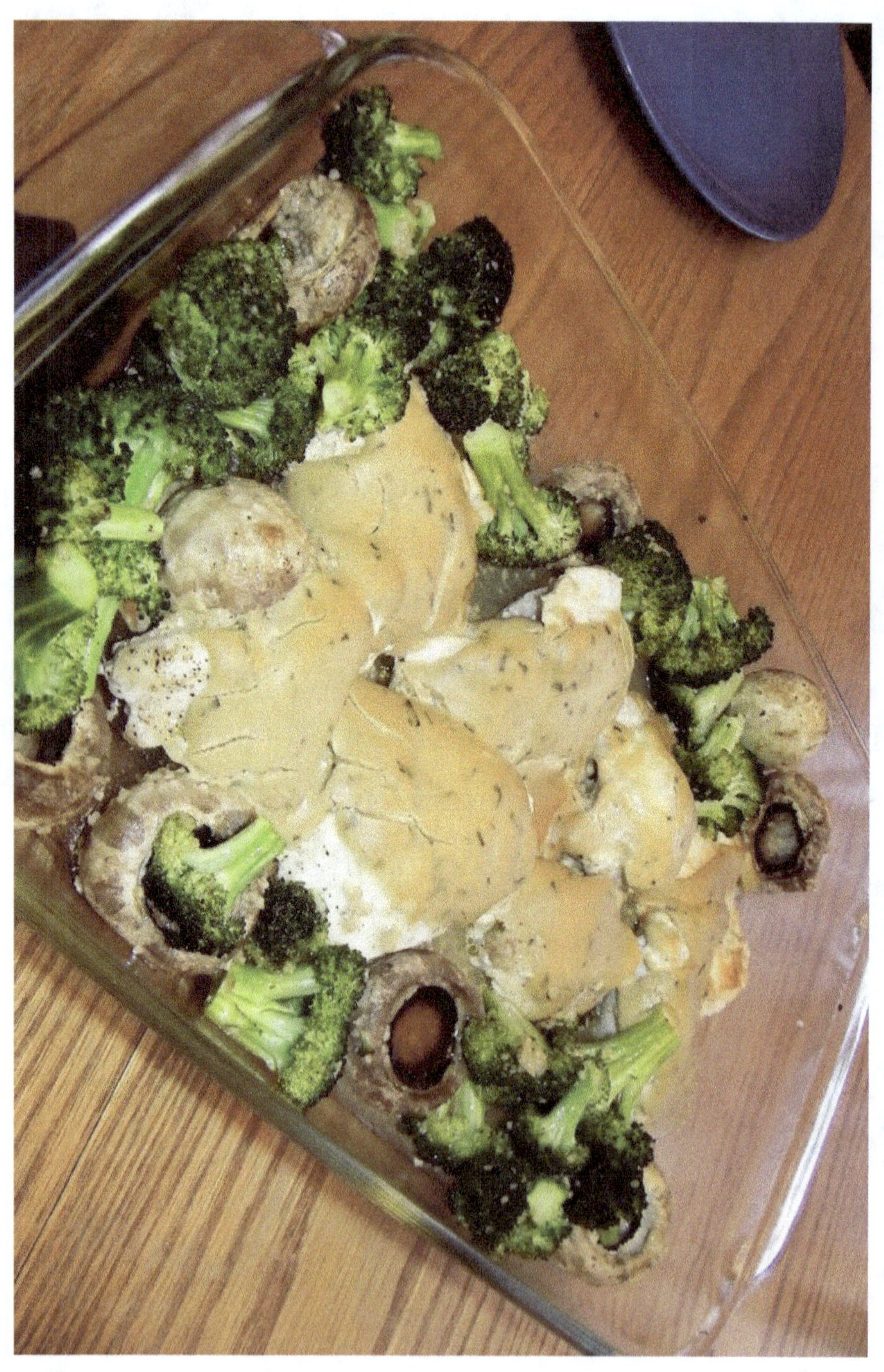

Rosemary Lemon Chicken

Servings: 4

Cooking Time: 14 Minutes

Ingredients:

- 1 kg chicken breast halves
- 1 lemon, peeled and sliced into rounds
- 1/2 orange, peeled and sliced into rounds, or to taste
- 3 cloves roasted garlic, or to taste
- salt and ground black pepper to taste
- 1 1/2 tablespoons olive oil, or to taste
- 1 1/2 teaspoons agave syrup, or to taste (optional)
- 1/4 cup water
- 2 sprigs fresh rosemary, stemmed, or to taste

Directions:

1.   Place chicken in the Instant Pot. Add lemon, orange, and garlic; season with salt and pepper. Drizzle olive oil and agave syrup (if using) on top. Add water and rosemary. Put the lid on the cooker and Lock in place.

2.   Select the "Meat" and "Stew" settings for High pressure, and cook for 14 minutes. Allow pressure to release naturally, about 20 minutes.

Nutrition Info: Calories 325 Fat 5 g Carbohydrates 20 g Sugar 2 g Protein 10 g Cholesterol 33 mg

Ginger Flavored Chicken

Servings: 6

Cooking Time: 15 Minutes

Ingredients:

- 1 kg boneless, skinless chicken breasts (frozen OR thawed)
- 6 tablespoons soy sauce
- 3 tablespoons rice vinegar
- 1/2 tablespoon honey
- 3 tablespoons water, broth, or orange juice
- 2 tablespoons chopped fresh ginger
- 6 cloves garlic, minced
- 3 teaspoons corn starch

Directions:

1. Place chicken breasts in Instant Pot.
2. In a small mixing bowl, whisk together: vinegar, soy sauce, honey, water, ginger and garlic. Pour mixture over chicken and coat evenly.

3. Secure lid on Instant Pot and cook at High pressure for 15 minutes. When the meat is cooked, release steam.

4. Remove chicken breasts and place on a cutting board. Bring remaining sauce in pan up to a simmer (use the Saute feature on an electric cooker). Combine cornstarch with 3 teaspoons cold water and then pour mixture into pan. Simmer until sauce is thickened and the turn off heat.

5. Shred chicken and return to pot with sauce.

Nutrition Info: Calories 313 Fat 25.6 g Carbohydrates 15.6 g Sugar 7 g Protein 8 g Cholesterol 36 mg

Crock-pot Slow Cooker Tex-mex Chicken

Servings: 6

Cooking Time: 4 Hours 40 Minutes

Ingredients:

- 4 tablespoons cup water
- 1 teaspoon ground cumin
- 1 lb boneless chicken thighs, visible fat removed, rinsed, and patted dry
- 1 (10 oz) can diced tomatoes and green chilies
- 1 (16 oz) package frozen onion and pepper strips, thawed

Directions:

1. Spray a skillet with cooking spray and turn heat flame on.
2. Place chicken thighs into the skillet and cook each side until browned over medium heat. Once browned, take out from the skillet.

3. To the same skillet, add peppers and onions and cook until tender.

4. Transfer cooked peppers and onions into 4- to 5-quart Crock-Pot slow cooker followed by chicken thighs on top.

5. Place tomatoes along with 4 tablespoons of water over chicken. Cook for about 4 hours on Low.

6. Add 1 teaspoon ground cumin and cook further for half an hour.

7. Once done, take it out and serve right away!

Nutrition Info: 121 calories; 3.2 g fat; 6.4 g total carbs; 16 g protein

Slow-cooker Chicken Fajita Burritos

Servings: 8

Cooking Time: 6 Hrs

Ingredients:

- 1 teaspoon cumin
- 1 cup cheddar cheese + 2 tablespoons reduced-fat, shredded
- 1 lb. chicken strips, skinless and boneless
- 8 large low-carb tortillas
- 1 green pepper, sliced
- 1 can (15 oz) black beans, rinsed and drained
- 1 red pepper, sliced
- 1/3 cup water
- 1 medium onion, sliced
- ½ cup salsa
- 1 tablespoon chili powder
- 1 teaspoon garlic powder

Directions:

1.   Place strips of chicken breast in a slow-cooker.
2.   Top chicken with all ingredients mentioned above except for cheese and tortillas. Cover the cooker and cook for approximately 6 hours, until done.
3.   Shred chicken with a fork.
4.   Serve half cup of chicken on each tortilla along with the bean mixture.
5.   Finish with 2 tablespoons of shredded cheese, then fold tortilla into a burrito.

Nutrition Info: 250 calories; 7 g fat; 31 g total carbs; 28 g protein

Chicken With Chickpeas

Servings: 4

Cooking Time: 36 Minutes

Ingredients:

- 2 tablespoons olive oil
- 1 pound skinless, boneless chicken breast, cubed
- 2 carrots, peeled and sliced
- 1 onion, chopped
- 2 celery stalks, chopped
- 2 garlic cloves, chopped
- 1 tablespoon fresh ginger root, minced
- ½ teaspoon dried oregano, crushed
- ¾ teaspoon ground cumin
- ½ teaspoon paprika
- ¼-13 teaspoon cayenne pepper
- ¼ teaspoon ground turmeric
- 1 cup tomatoes, crushed
- 1½ cups low-sodium chicken broth

- 1 zucchini, sliced
- 1 cup boiled chickpeas, drained
- 1 tablespoon fresh lemon juice

Directions:

1. In a large nonstick pan, heat the oil over medium heat and cook the chicken cubes for about 4-5 minutes.
2. With a slotted spoon, transfer the chicken cubes onto a plate.
3. In the same pan, add the carrot, onion, celery and garlic and sauté for about 4-5 minutes.
4. Add the ginger, oregano and spices and sauté for about 1 minute.
5. Add the chicken, tomato and broth and bring to a boil.
6. Now, reduce the heat to low and simmer for about 10 minutes.
7. Add the zucchini and chickpeas and simmer, covered for about 15 minutes.
8. Stir in the lemon juice and serve hot.

9. Meal Prep Tip: Transfer the chicken mixture into a large bowl and set aside to cool. Divide the mixture into 4 containers evenly. Cover the containers and refrigerate for 1-2 days. Reheat in the microwave before serving.

Nutrition Info: Calories 308 Total Fat 12.3 g Saturated Fat 2.7 g Cholesterol 66 mg Total Carbs 19 g Sugar 5.3g Fiber 4.7 g Sodium 202 mg Potassium 331 mg Protein 30.7 g